PATIENT'S GUIDE TO THE BIONIC EYE

I0493962

Jeffrey N. Weiss, M.D.

FOR ALL OUR PATIENTS

PATIENT'S GUIDE TO THE BIONIC EYE

WHAT IS THE BIONIC EYE?

While the term "bionic eye" captures the imagination, a more accurate phrase would be "retinal prosthesis" or "retinal implant." This is a medical device which is being added to a portion of the retina that is still viable. None of the devices discussed can replace the retina and they cannot be used when the retina is completely nonfunctional. In this booklet, I will attempt to discuss the reality of how these devices work, what they actually do, and what they hope to do in the future.

WHO IS THIS BOOK FOR?

This book will typically be read by the family member or friend of someone with a degenerative retinal disease that has already lost vision. I have attempted to present the information in a balanced fashion. I have no financial relationships with any of the companies discussed.

HOW DOES THE EYE WORK?

Simplistically, the eye has been compared to a camera. The cornea and lens of the eye focus light onto the retina, or the "film in the camera." The optic nerve carries the image to the brain, like a cable to a computer monitor, for interpretation.

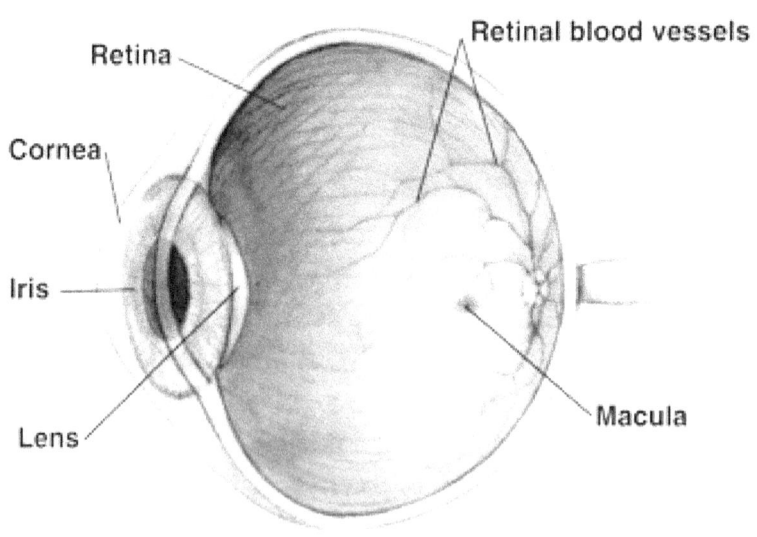

Retina

Retinal blood vessels

Cornea

Iris

Lens

Macula

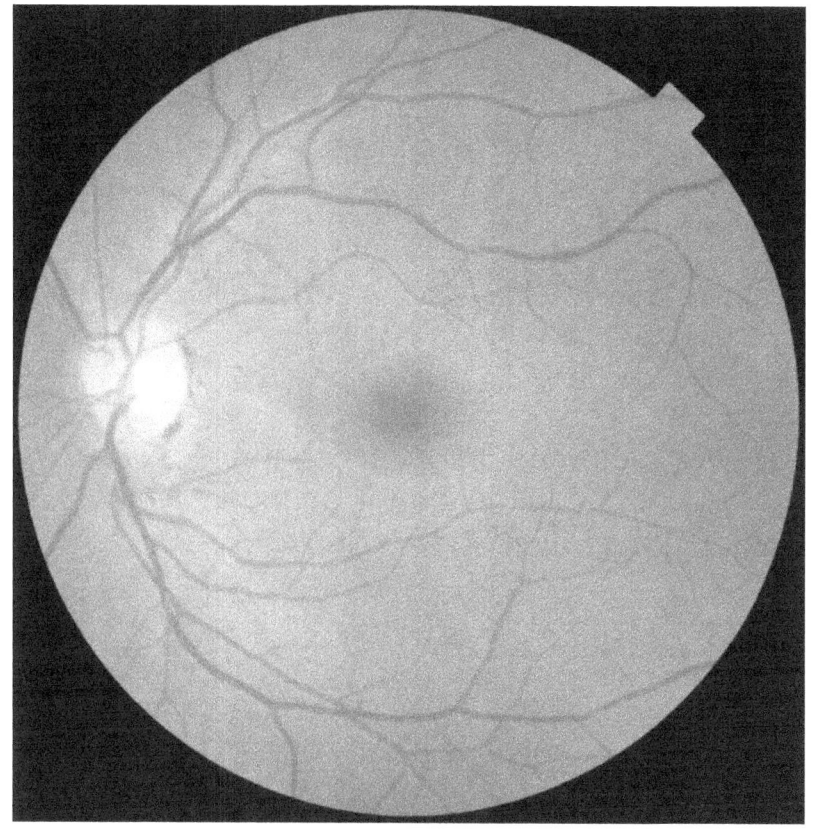

This is what your physician see when he looks into your left eye with an ophthalmoscope. The optic disc is the circular object on the left, the macula is the reddish structure in the middle of the photograph. The fovea is the slightly clearer object in the center of the macula. The retinal veins are slightly wider and deeper in color than the arteries. In your right eye, the location of the optic disc and the macula would be reversed; the optic nerve would be on the right side of the photo and the macula on the left side.

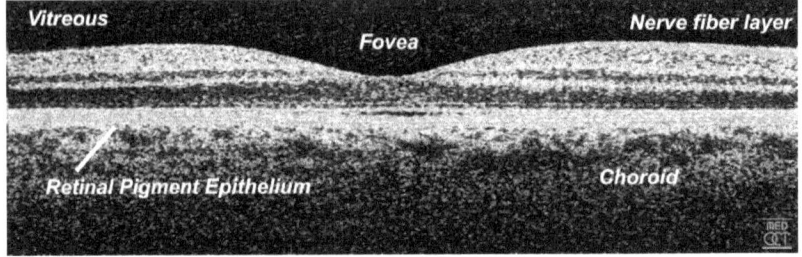

This is a picture of an optical coherence tomogram (OCT), an examination test which demonstrates a cross-sectional view of the retina.

Our retina actually consists of 10 layers. Starting inside the eye, moving backwards or posteriorly they are:

1. Inner limiting membrane - basement membrane made by Muller cells.

2. Nerve fiber layer - this layer represents the axons, similar to "wires" coming from the ganglion layer below. The nerve fiber layer forms the optic nerve and transmits messages to the brain.

3. Ganglion cell layer - this layer contains the nuclei of the ganglion cells and some amacrine cells.

4. Inner plexiform layer - contains the connection, or synapse between the bipolar cell axons and the connection structures, or dendrites of the ganglion and amacrine cells.

5. Inner nuclear layer - contains the nuclei and the cell bodies of the bipolar cells.

6. Outer plexiform layer - the ends of the rods and cones (the photoreceptors) make synapses, or connections with the dendrites of the bipolar cells.

7. Outer nuclear layer - contains the cell bodies of the rods and cones.

8. External limiting membrane - separates the inner segment of the photoreceptors from their cell nucleus.

9. Photoreceptor layer - contains the rods and cones.

10.   Retinal pigment epithelium - a layer of cells.

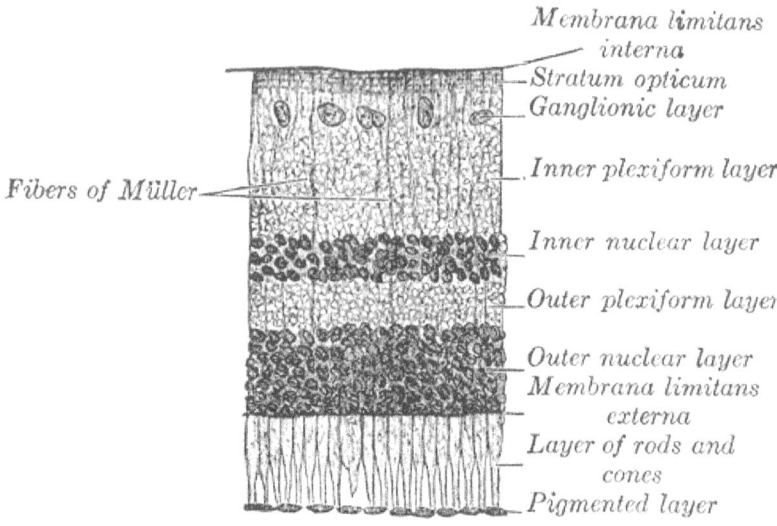

Membrana limitans interna
Stratum opticum
Ganglionic layer

Inner plexiform layer

Fibers of Müller

Inner nuclear layer

Outer plexiform layer

Outer nuclear layer
Membrana limitans externa
Layer of rods and cones
Pigmented layer

The retina and optic nerve are part of the central nervous system (CNS) and are the only parts of the CNS that can be directly visualized. The image you see is not just displayed on the retina, it is processed in the retina. In this respect the retina is more like a computer than a simple film in a camera.

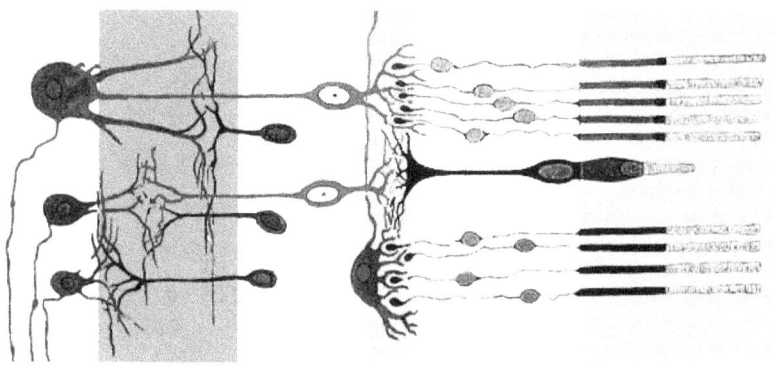

Light passes from the left (the front of the retina) through the nerve layers to reach the rods and the cones on the far right. A chemical change occurs in the rods and cones which sends a signal to the nerves. The signal is processed by the bipolar and horizontal cells (yellow layer), to the amacrine cells and ganglion cells (purple layer), and then to the optic nerve fibers which go to the brain.

The retina contains approximately 7 million cones, and 75 - 150 million rods. The cones are utilized in daylight, and for color vision, the rods in dim light and black and white vision. The human eye contains one fovea, the depression in the retina in charge of sharp central vision. The fovea is dominated by cones, the peripheral retina by rods. (Certain birds, like hawks, actually contain two foveas.) While you are reading this book you are using your central vision, if someone walks into the room you will be aware of this by the stimulation of your peripheral vision.

Since there are 100 times the number of retinal receptors as there are nerve fibers in the optic nerve, a large amount of signal processing must be performed in the retina. The most accurate information is provided by the fovea, which although it represents less than 2 degrees of visual angle, is connected to 10% of the axons of the optic nerve.

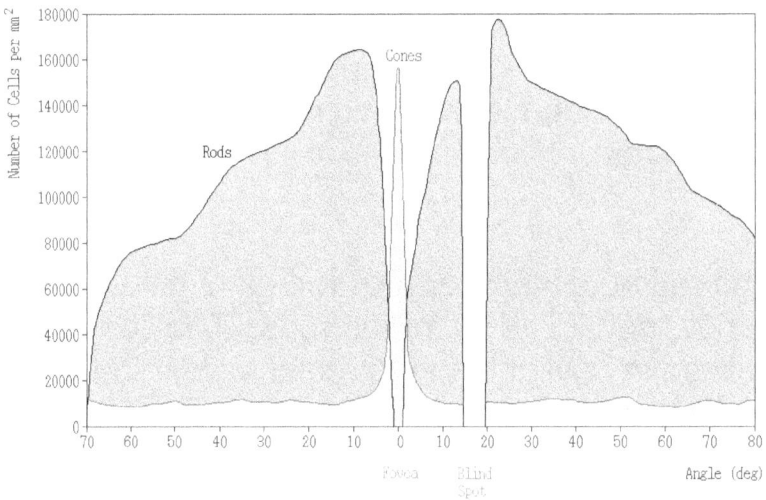

In order to compress the image to fit the optic nerve capacity the bipolar and ganglion cells perform "center surround processing." There are "on" and "off" centers. "On" centers are positively weighted in the center and negatively weighted around the center. "Off" centers are the opposite. They function similar to a mathematical algorithm in enhancing the edges of an image.

	On center cell	Off center cell
Light on center only	Ganglion cell fires rapidly	Ganglion cell does not fire
Light on surround only	Cell does not fire	Cell fires rapidly
No light on center or surround	Cell does not fire	Cell does not fire
Light on center and surround	Weak response (low frequency firing)	Weak response (low frequency firing)

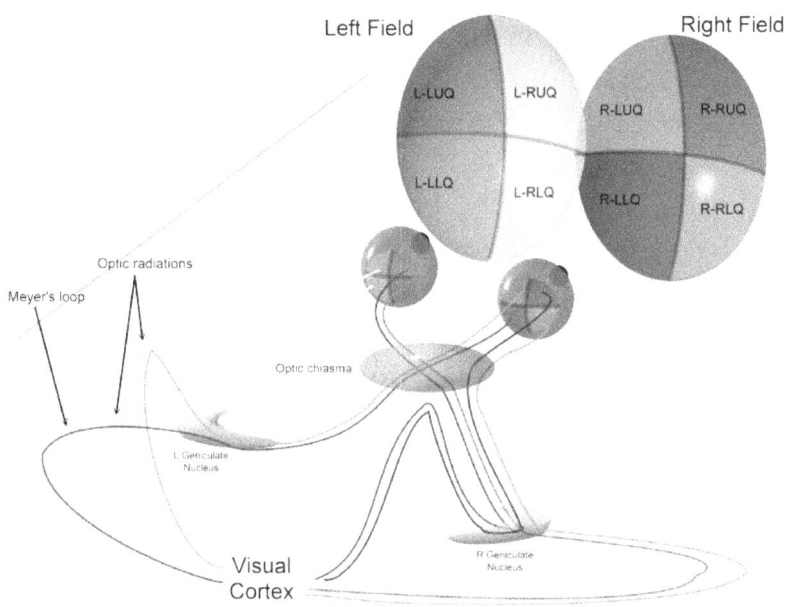

L/R - LUQ Left/Right Eye - Left Upper Quadrant

L/R - LLQ Left/Right Eye - Left Lower Quadrant

L/R - RUQ Left/Right Eye - Right Upper Quadrant

L/R - RLQ Left/Right Eye - Right Lower Quadrant

The encoded image is sent via the axons of the ganglion cells through the nerve and optic chiasm to the lateral geniculate nucleus (LGN). The output of the LGN is transmitted to the visual cortex of the brain.

This discussion is not meant to be a detailed analysis of retinal function, but to serve as an example of the complexity of sight.

Patient's ask me why I can't just give them a new eye. You now have an idea why this would be impossible at the present time. The eye is directly connected to the brain by tissue that we cannot regenerate. Perhaps one day, but not now.

****

The ocular implants that are presently available are all designed for conditions affecting the rod and cone photoreceptors, such as retinitis pigmentosa. In these conditions the inner retina remains intact. This means that these devices cannot be used in patients blind from retinal detachment, glaucoma, or any condition where retinal layers, other than the photoreceptor layers, are affected.

With this in mind, now let us explore what is being done with the bionic eye, prosthetic retina, or retinal implant.

At the present time, there are more than 20 groups working on bionic eyes.

Traditional eye charts to measure visual acuity are difficult to apply in situations of very low, or poor vision. Grating visual acuity, motion detection, ambulation, orientation, letter identification, electrically elicited visual evoked potentials (eVEPs), etc. are all being explored in order to quantitate improvements in vision seen with retinal prosthetics.

WHAT ARE THE IMPORTANT CRITERIA TO LOOK FOR?

1. Clinical Availability - How far along are they?

2. Vision Restoration Potential - Clinical improvement in patient's vision.

   External cameras relay images to electrodes. Photodiode arrays are directly stimulated by the light. Features affecting visual performance following implantation are: interfacing with the remaining functional retina, pixel number, and density and field of vision.

3. Long Term Biocompatibility - Long term risk of infection, exposure.

   Will the implant continue to work over time? Will the retina lose sensitivity?

4. Learning - Can the implant be personalized for the patient?

I will discuss the most promising approaches.

1. Second-Sight Medical Products Inc. (Sylmar, CA)

Their unit, the Argus 2, is both approved in the U.S. (FDA) and the European Union (CE) for treating end stage retinitis pigmentosa. This condition affects more than 1 million people worldwide, or approximately 1 in 4,000 people. More than 70 patients have been implanted with this device, 35 since it received FDA approval. The patient must have an intact optic nerve and reasonably intact inner retinal architecture.

This device is an epiretinal implant consisting of a 60 electrode array, 200 microns in diameter. Epiretinal means placement on the surface of the retina. A vitrectomy (the removal of the vitreous body within the eye) is first performed. The device is tacked in place on top of the nerve fibers of the retinal ganglion cells by a plastic tack that extends from the retina to the sclera. The epiretinal device is not light sensitive. Wires lead from the implant through a small hole in the sclera to a receiver that is located on a band outside the eye. The receiver is covered by tissue so it is not exposed to the outside environment.

There is an external camera (510 x 492 pixel resolution) mounted on a pair of spectacles powered by a battery powered computer, that transmits the image via an antenna to the receiver on the eye. The device is not to be implanted bilaterally, but only in the worse seeing eye.

In the initial study, 30 patients that were blind, or with bare light perception secondary to retinitis pigmentosa were implanted with the Argus 2. After surgery, all the patients could perceive light. In order to determine the effectiveness of the device testing was done with it switched on, then off. When the implant was turned on, patients performed statistically better in object localization (96% of patients), motion discrimination (57%), and discrimination of oriented gratings (23%) with an estimated visual field of 20 degrees. Patients were able to identify doors and posts while walking. The best recorded visual acuity was 20/1260.

70% of the patients implanted did not have any serious adverse events.
More than 50 patients have been living with the device for more than 6 years. Only one of the 30 patients in the initial clinical trial had the device removed.

NOTE

The standard Snellen eye chart you see in an ophthalmologist's office is set at a 20 foot distance (the numerator or top number of the 20/1260) and the largest letter on this eye chart, the "E" is 400. If you can only see the large "E" at 20 feet, your vision is recorded as 20/400. Obviously, the 1260 letter is quite large. But, any improvement in a blind patient is an incredible accomplishment.

Initially, the retinal implant surgery took more than 3.8 hours to perform. With further experience, operative time decreased to 1.8 hours. The number of significant adverse events also decreased with further implantation experience. The Argus system implant, the surgical procedure and follow-up is estimated to cost approximately $115,000. Since there is no other treatment for functionally blind patients with retinitis pigmentosa, insurance companies are expected to cover the cost.

In a study reported in the British Journal of Ophthalmology in 2013, 29 patients with retinitis pigmentosa, and one with choroideremia with light perception vision underwent implantation of the prosthesis. Two patients were subsequently excluded from the study; one had the device explanted (removed) as it eroded through the overlying conjunctiva, the other patient had a retinal detachment.

21 of the remaining 28 patients took part in a letter and word reading study. A subgroup of six subjects was able to consistently read small letters, (0.9 cm (1.7 degree) at 30 cm, and four subjects correctly identified unrehearsed two, three, and four letter words. The average implant duration was almost 20 months. This is an excellent achievement in almost blind patients, who, prior to the development of this device, had no hope for improvement. It is important to note that the average time to correctly identify letters took from 6 to 221 seconds.

SOME OTHER THINGS TO NOTE

If you have your natural lens in your eye, it will be removed during the implant surgery.

Contraindications to having the implant surgery include: optic nerve disease, central retinal artery or vein occlusion, retinal detachment, trauma, severe strabismus, corneal opacity.

Having any metallic or active implanted device in the head, i.e., cochlear implant, is contraindicated. After implantation, there are permanent restrictions on the use of certain types of MRI, and other electromagnetic and ultrasound procedures.

Eye rubbing can cause significant problems following the procedure.

For further information you may visit ClinicalTrials.gov NCT00407602. The study has a primary completion date of March, 2012, and an estimated study completion date of August, 2019.

THE ARGUS 2 EPIRETINAL IMPLANT

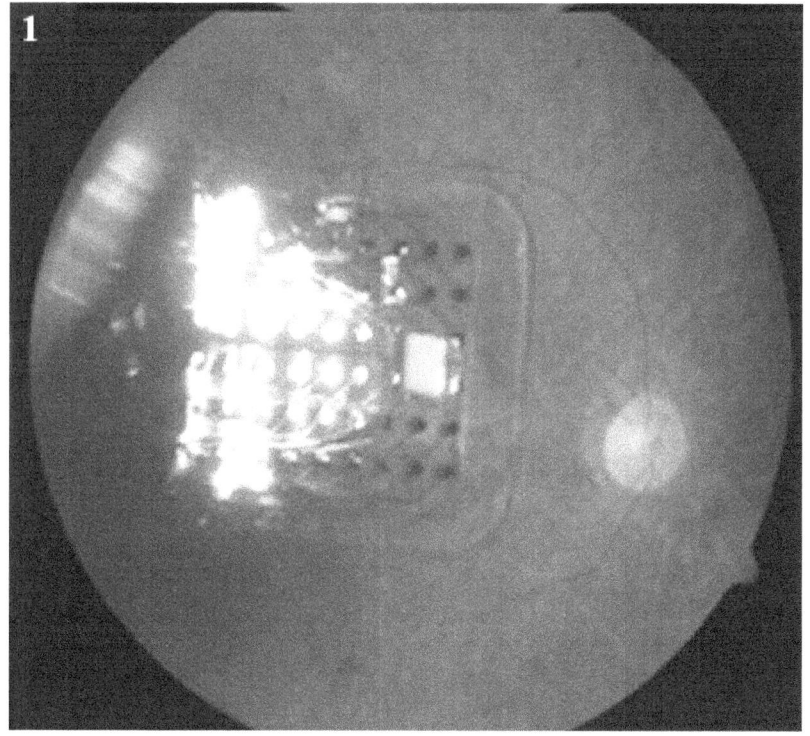

SURGERY LOCATIONS

CALIFORNIA

Doheny Eye Institute, Los Angeles

University of California, San Francisco

MARYLAND

Johns Hopkins, Wilmer Eye Institute, Baltimore

NEW YORK

Columbia University, Department of Ophthalmology, Edward S. Harkness Eye Institute, New York, New York

PENNSYLVANIA

University of Pennsylvania, Scheie Eye Institute, Philadelphia

Wills Eye Hospital, Philadelphia

TEXAS

Retina Foundation of the Southwest, Dallas

FRANCE

Centre d'Investigation Clinique, Service d'Ophtalmologie, Quinze-Vingts National Eye Hospital, Paris

MEXICO

Puerto de Hierro, Centro Medico, Centro de Retina, Zapopan, Jalisco

SWITZERLAND

Clinique d'Ophthalmologie Hopitaux, Universitaires de Geneve, Geneva

UNITED KINGDOM

Moorfields Eye Hospital, Vitreoretinal Research Unit, London

Manchester Royal Eye Hospital, Manchester

****

ALPHA IMS IMPLANT

The Alpha IMS Implant is manufactured by Retina Implant AG (Reutlingen, Germany). It is CE approved and is under review by the FDA as an "Investigational Device."

The implant is placed under the retina (subretinal). The implant consists of 1500 photodiodes. It is light sensitive. The patient carries a small box that wirelessly provides the power for the device. There is a transmitter antenna that is placed under the skin behind the ear (subdermal) and kept in place by a magnet. A cable runs from the subdermal receiver to the eye. The implant chip is inserted through a flap cut into the sclera and advanced beneath the fovea of the retina as subfoveal placement was shown to be superior in outcomes compared to para (near) or nonfoveal placement. The implant absorbs photons of light and converts them into an electrical signal for the bipolar retinal cell layer to process. The 1500 photodiodes are 15 x 30 microns in size. The intraocular dimensions of the implant are 3.1 mm x 3.0 mm x 70 microns.

The length of the subdermal cable to the power control unit is 22 mm.

In the initial study, 11 patients received a wire-bound implant, the next 9 patients received a wireless device. The implant covers approximately 15 degree of the visual field. Of the 9 patients, light perception was restored in 8/9 patients, light localization (7/9), motion detection (5/9), grating acuity (6/9) and visual acuity was measured up to 20/546 (2/9). Identification, localization, and discrimination of objects statistically improved in repeated tests over a 9 month period.

NOTE

Despite the fact that the Retina Implant AG has 1500 electrodes, versus the Argus 2, 60 electrodes, a 2013 French article stated that patient visual performances were fairly similar with each device.

They also describe the challenges in increasing pixel density corresponding to an increase in electrode number and density. Challenges include, stimulation modality, tissue/implant interface design, electrode materials, and the visual information encoder. Another 2012 article pointed out that implanted retinal electronics must keep power dissipation low to stay below the microglial thermal damage threshold.

Further information may be found at
ClinicalTrials.gov NCT01024803,
NCT00515814.

RETINA IMPLANT AG SUBRETINAL IMPLANT

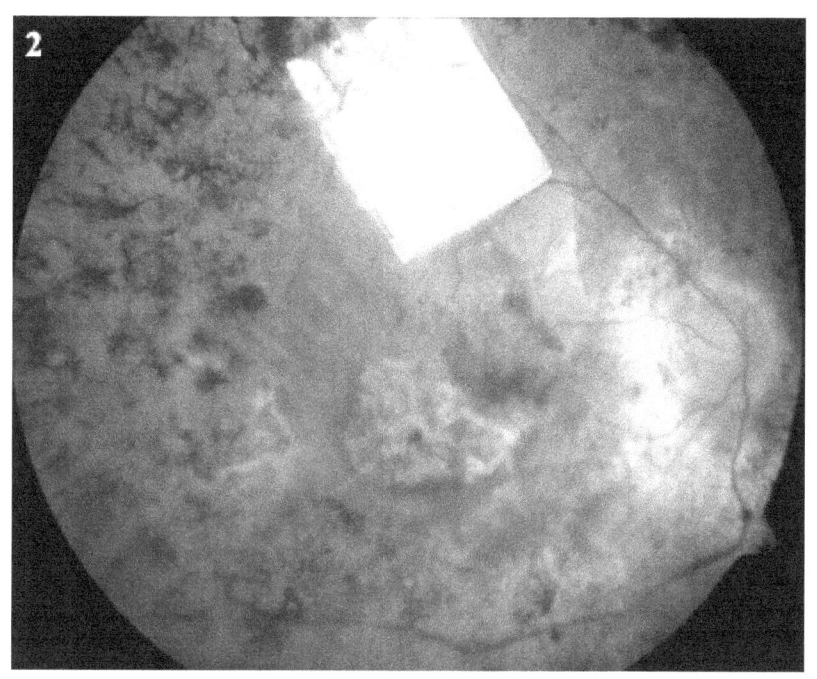

SURGERY LOCATIONS

GERMANY

Helmut Sachs, MD, PD, Dresden
Contact: Ursula Brunner   +49 351 480 1830
brunner@eye-regensburg.de

Claus Eckardt, MD, Prof., Frankfurt-Hoechst
Contact: Ute Reissig, MD   +49 69 3106 2972
C.Eckardt@em.uni-frankfurt.de

Johann Roider, MD, Prof., Kiel
Contact: Jost Hillenkamp, MD, PD +49 431 597
2402 jhillenkamp@ophthalmol.uni-kiel.de

Karl-Ulrich Bartz-Schmidt, MD, Prof., Tuebingen
Contact: Barbara Wilhelm, MD, Prof +49 70
71298 48 98 barbara.wilhelm@stz-biomed.de
Contact: Anusch Hekmat, PhD +49 7121 36403
ext 251 a.hekmat@retina-implant.de

HUNGARY

Miklos Resch, MD, PhD, Budapest
Contact: Akos Kusnyerik, MD +36 20 922 00 04
kusnyerik@yahoo.com

ITALY

Stanislao Rizzo, MD, Pisa
Contact: Emanuele Di Bartolo, MD +39 50
992175 emadibar@tin.it

UNITED KINGDOM

Timothy L Jackson, MB, ChB, PhD, London
Contact: Barbara Kolator   +44 20 3299 1297
Barbara.Kolator@kch.nhs.uk

Robert MacLaren, MD, Prof., DPhil, DipEd, Oxford
Contact: Robert MacLaren, MD +44 1865 234782 robert.maclaren@eye.ox.ac.uk
Contact: Susan Downes, MD susan.downes@orh.nhs.uk

****

PILOT STUDY OF A SUPRACHOROIDAL RETINAL PROSTHESIS

ClinicalTrials.gov Identifier - NCT01603576

Sponsor - Center for Eye Research Australia

This study is ongoing, but not recruiting participants.

Eligibility Criteria - Outer retinal degenerative disease such as retinitis pigmentosa or choroideremia.

Investigators -

Study Director - Anthony Burkitt, PhD
Bionic Vision Australia

Principal Investigator - Robyn Guymer, MBBS, PhD Centre for Eye Research Australia

Estimated Enrollment - 10 patients

Study Start Date - May 2012

Estimated Primary Completion Date - May 2015

There is limited information about this work. The suprachoroidal implant is inserted through a tunnel in the sclera from the back of the eye. The electrodes sit between the sclera and the choroid and do not touch the retina.

Why a suprachoroidal implant? To answer this question let us look at some of the potential problems of the other 2 implants.

1. Epiretinal Implant - The risks of this type of implant are: surgical trauma, poor implant fixation, retinal damage due to uneven pressure from the implant and retinal detachment.

2. Subretinal Implant - The risks of this type of implant include: photoreceptor loss, damage to the inner retina, disruption of the retinal pigment epithelium and surgical trauma including retinal tears. There is a greater difficulty in surgical implantation and a limit to the size of the implant.

The potential benefits of a suprachoroidal implant are: the surgery is safer than that needed for insertion of an epiretinal or subretinal implant (although there is a greater risk of bleeding).

There would be a much lower chance of damage to the neural retina.

Since nearly 70% of the variance in walking speed in patients with retinitis pigmentosa is accounted for the size of the visual field and contrast sensitivity, it would be beneficial to increase the size of the visual field. As previously mentioned, the visual field with the Argus 2 is approximately 20 degree and with the Retina Implant AG 15 degree. The size of the implant is limited when placed epi or subretinally but may be made larger when placed suprachoroidally. But a potential downside of this type of implant is that the threshold for retinal stimulation is higher than that required with an epiretinal or subretinal implant because the implant is located further away from inner retina.

A suprachoroidal implant was reported having been implanted in 7 cats. The implant was well tolerated for the 3 month study duration. Electrical stimulation of the implant at 2 weeks post implantation demonstrated a significant increase in signal which returned to baseline at 3 months

****

EPI-RET 3

This device is a fully intraocular epiretinal implant undergoing clinical testing in Europe. Six subjects were implanted for 28 days each. When the devices were removed, some of the tacks used to secure the implant were found to be loose and the growth of epiretinal membranes (scar) was observed. When patients were re-examined 2 years later, epiretinal membranes were observed at the tack site, but they did not cause patient symptoms.

Like the Argus 2 implant, a camera is mounted on eyeglasses, but unlike the Argus 2, the receiver is intraocular and replaces the patient's lens. A cable connects the receiver module to the 25 electrode epiretinal array. With no extraocular cable, the theoretical risk of serious adverse events may be lower. The 25 electrodes are 100 microns in diameter and the dimensions of the intraocular implant are 40 mm x 3 mm x 10 microns.

****

INTELLIGENT MEDICAL IMPLANTS

This epiretinal implant is in clinical trials in Europe. In one study, 3 patients were implanted with a 49 electrode array for 30 months. In the most recent study 20 patients were temporarily implanted for 45 minutes. The device uses an external camera with wireless data and power transfer. The receiver module connects to the epiretinal array via a cable through a scleral tunnel. The 49 electrodes are 100 - 360 microns in diameter and the implant dimensions are 60 mm x 1 mm x 10 microns.

What makes this device exciting is that it incorporates a retina encoder which allows the patient to individually calibrate the device so as to optimize their visual perceptions to match physical reality.

****

BOSTON RETINAL IMPLANT PROJECT

This is a subretinal implant that is not yet in human trials. The 100 electrode array has been implanted in two minipigs for 3 and for 5 months, respectively. Electrical stimulation demonstrated that the implant was functional. The 100 electrodes are 400 microns in diameter and the dimensions of the device are 5 mm x 10 microns. The extraocular dimensions of the electronic case are 11 x 11 x 2 mm in size.

****

NOTES

Electronic vision is different from normal vision. Patients report blurred borders and flickering vision. Both the rods and cones have a repetitive frequency. Repetitive stimulation by an electronic array may produce fading of an image.

The current electrode size has a theoretical maximum resolution of approximately 12 arc minutes whereas normal human vision can resolve one arc minute. Cones are only a few microns in diameter, make multiple connections with the inner retinal cells, and are in high concentration at the fovea. Contrast sensitivity at low luminance is difficult due to the loss of the on/off system (discussed above) in retinitis pigmentosa. Current implants are estimated to provide approximately 15% of normal contrast.

There are 3 types of cones for distinguishing colors. As the electrode size is much greater than the size of the cone, patients with epiretinal arrays have reported color vision, but the colors are related to the area stimulated and not the color of the viewed object. Patients receiving the subretinal implants have reported greyish images, with a slight yellowish tinge. The subretinal arrays are probably stimulating all 3 cone types at one time, preventing distinct color vision.

Possible alternative approaches to electronic implant arrays include Stem Cell Surgery and Gene Replacement Surgery. For more information on these two topics, I have written "Patient's Guide to Retinal and Optic Nerve Stem Cell Surgery" and "Patient's Guide to Retinal Gene Therapy." Both books are available on Amazon.